Teenage girls With Acne Problem

...Discover Proven Methods To Actually Cure Your Acne for Life

---

By

JEROME N. OHANA

NATURO-THERAPIST
CERTIFIED

Disclaimer

The information contained in this eBook is offered for informational purposes solely, and it is geared towards providing exact and reliable information in regards to the topic and issue covered. The author and the publisher does not warrant that the information contained in this e-book is fully complete and shall not be responsible for any errors or omissions.

The author and publisher shall have neither liability nor responsibility to any person or entity concerning any reparation, damages, or monetary loss caused or alleged to be caused directly or indirectly by this e-book. Therefore, this eBook should be used as a guide - not as the ultimate source.

The publication is sold with the idea that the publisher is not required to render accounting, officially permitted, or otherwise, qualified services. If advice is necessary, legal or professional, a practiced individual in the profession should be ordered.

CONTENTS

Introduction

Approximately 85% of teenage girls in the world are going to battle acne. Girls, in particular, are susceptible to the detrimental toll it takes on their self-esteem.

During puberty, girls already have a plethora of development and emotional issues to deal with. The changes they experience while going from girls to women are for many, so numerous and rapid that they barely have time to come to terms with them.

Menstruation and the accompanying hormone increase can be a big challenge for teen girls. Add to that some of the other physical changes, such as growth spurts, body development, and hair growing in new places, and you have the makings of a problematic situation. Add acne to that already challenging mix, and it can be, for some girls, an emotional roller coaster ride.

Girls are faced with the most excellent possibility of developing acne pimples during puberty. Because of the increase in hormone levels, adolescence can be a stressful time for them. They may have mood swings, and can sometimes be irritable.

The onset of acne only serves to heighten the possibility that their self-esteem will be affected. It can be an obstacle for even the most capable and confident of girls.

Usually, through the age of puberty, the body's endocrine typicoperates again, then the irritating acne disappears. However, most girls are not patient enough to wait before ageing acne; those girls then squeeze the new acne out by hand.

Furthermore, no cleaning the skin often will lead to acne infections. Meanwhile, more acne will be swelling, rotting and then become very dangerous boils.

Acne isn't something that is normal or is to be expected. It isn't something that we should have to deal with. Acne is a sign that something inside of us has gone wrong. The overabundance of hormones in our systems is what's causing the acne in the first place. But if everything were working as it was supposed to be, our body would be able to get rid of these hormones promptly, avoiding any further problems.

Natural remedies have been around for ages and have been proven effective to cure illnesses or different types of diseases, including skin diseases like acne. If you are suffering from acne for a long time, now you probably have tried almost everything without success. This book contains thorough pieces of advice for acne using natural methods as an alternative remedy.

Let's get started!

Basic Knowledge of The Skin

The skin is not just the body's wrapper. While it's true that the skin is the outermost layer between you and your environment, it is much more than just a simple cover for your bones and organs. The skin is the largest organ of the body. You may not think of the skin as an organ, but it is, and it plays an essential role in overall health.

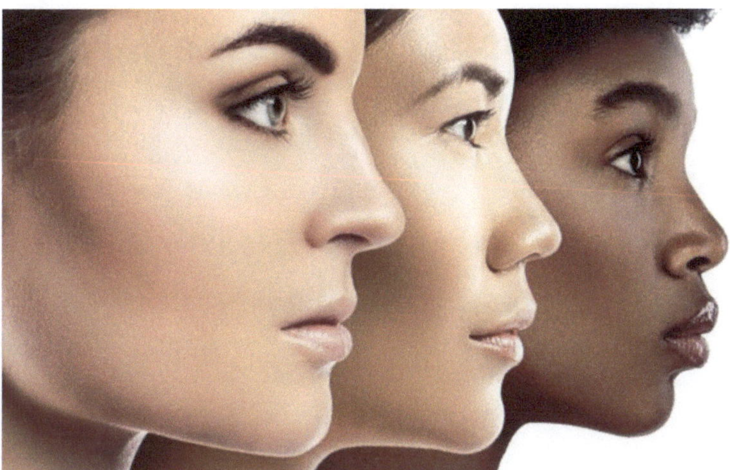

Not only does our outer shell encase us, but it also serves many significant functions including:

- Protecting us from injury and parasite invasion;

- Providing us with our sense of touch;

- Regulating our body temperature and preventing dehydration;

- Aiding in detoxification and elimination;

- Assisting with vitamin d synthesis when it's exposed to sunlight;

- Helping our immune system fight infection.

Yes, the importance of our skin goes way beyond wrinkles and age spots. Our surface comprises an intricate array of cells and systems that work together to keep us vibrant and healthy while contributing to our overall wellness.

Our skin is alive and dynamic. It is always changing and regenerating itself, though at different rates, depending on our age. Infants regenerate skin cells in as few as fourteen days. By the time we reach middle age, it can take about thirty-five days to generate new skin cells. On average, the life cycle of a skin cell is twenty-eight days. The skin grows faster than any other organ in the body. At this moment, your skin is creating, growing, and regenerating millions of new skin cells.

There are two distinct layers of the skin:

- The epidermis, or the outer layer

- The dermis

The dermis, which is located just under what we refer to like the skin, contains the nerves that give us the ability to feel changes in our environment, including heat, cold, pain and pressure, plus the sensation associated with touch. The dermis also connects blood vessels to the base of the epidermis.

Most skin cell activity and metamorphosis take place in the skin's outer layer, the epidermis. There are five layers within the dermis. Specialized skin cells work their way up from the bottom layer to the top.

One of the critical roles of the skin is to protect us from our external environment. Our skin defends us from injury, environmental assault, parasites, and other foreign invaders.

The skin is one of the most sophisticated sponges ever created. That's why it's vital to protect it and take care of it.

Types Of Human Skin

Human skin is a real organ that allows the interaction of the internal environment of our body with the world around us. It communicates with the outside world sending and receiving an infinite number of messages and signals.

It acts as a real barrier and prevents the passage of foreign substances and the release of other useful materials. It also behaves as a place of exchange and intercommunication with the outside world, sending to our organism many valuable messages from the external environment.

The various types of skin, along with hair and eye colour, are divided into six classes, which differ from each other for the manner of response to the amount of solar radiation that they receive. These types are:

1. Very light skin, blue eyes, blond or red hair: often burn, occasionally tans.
2. Light skin, light eye and hair colour: often burns and tans with difficulty.
3. Intermediate light skin, brown or green eyes, brown hair: rarely burns, usually tans with a golden hue.
4. Intermediate dark or "olive" skin, dark eyes and nose: burns rarely, often tans.
5. Dark or brown skin, dark eyes and nose: naturally brown leather.
6. Very dark skin: typically black, brown skin.

Acne Definitions

I s there any difference between a pimple and a whitehead? How do you tell a papule from a pustule? The following list of definitions can help teen girls find out what all those skincare terms mean and learn more about treating acne pimples.

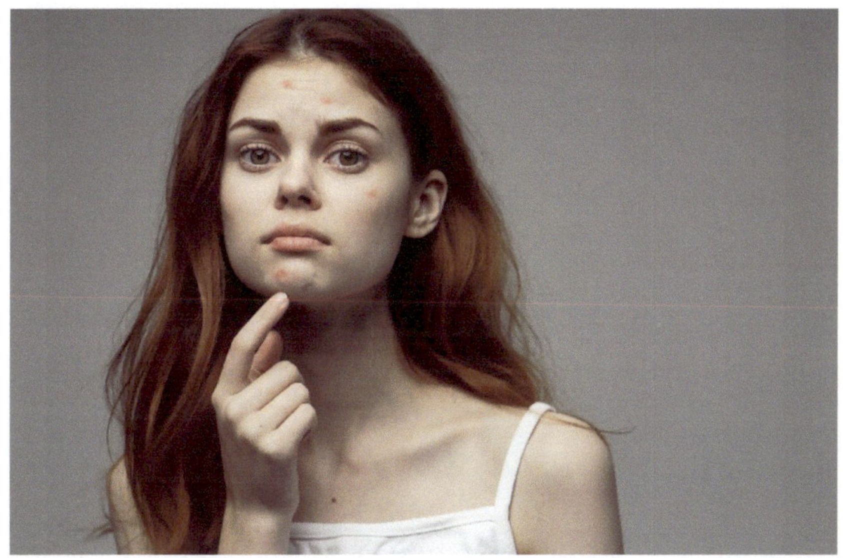

— Acne

A skin disorder than ranges in seriousness from mild to severe and affects nearly 80% of those from 12 to 22. It's caused when male hormones trigger the overproduction of oil from the sebaceous glands in the hair follicles. Dead cells that trap the oil can block these follicles.

Bacteria grow in this environment, causing the pimples. These various lesions are the primary symptom of acne.

— Acne Vulgaris

The general medical term for common acne, which is defined as the appearance of one or more blackheads, whiteheads, papules or pustules.

— Androgens

Hormones which, in addition to various other functions in the body, stimulate oil production in the follicles; because they are typically present at higher levels in males than females, it is common for males to have more severe acne.

— Benzoyl Peroxide

A common ingredient in topical acne medications; benzoyl peroxide has oxidative properties which destroy acne-causing bacteria.

— Blackhead

A non-inflamed acne lesion that is the result of pores becoming clogged with oils and dead skin cells; blackheads appear as small, tightly-packed, darkened pores.

— Comedones

Blackheads and whiteheads, the least severe type of acne, are referred to collectively as comedones. They are the result of pores becoming clogged with dead skin cells, hair, and skin oils; a whitehead results when the pore is closed, while open comedones are known as blackheads.

— Cyst

These are broad, deep and painful acne lesions: the most severe type of wound. Cysts can cause extensive and permanent scarring if not successfully treated.

Cystic acne may call for more intensive treatment than more moderate forms, including antibiotics and stronger topical medications. A dermatologist is almost certainly required to deal with this severe and inflammatory acne adequately.

— Follicle

Minute openings in the skin through which hairs grow; they also contain glands which secrete oils necessary for keeping the skin lubricated.

— Hormones

Numerous chemicals that govern a wide range of processes in the body, including oil production in the skin. When these hormones are present at elevated levels, excess oil production occurs, often leading to clogged pores.

— Icepick Scar

A deep, jagged-edged scar caused by severe acne.

— Keloid

A raised scar that covers more area than the original wound or blemish.

— Macule

A flat, red or darkened patch of skin that results from a healed acne lesion; macules may be present for several weeks after the original blemish has healed.

─ **Nodule**

A hardened, painful lump in the skin that occurs when the follicle wall is damaged due to inflammation from an acne lesion.

─ **Noncomedogenic**

A substance that is unlikely to cause acne; look for noncomedogenic cleansers and cosmetics to avoid the appearance of acne on your skin.

─ **Papule**

A small, inflamed, red bump on the surface of the skin.

─ **P. acnes**

Short for Propionibacterium acnes, the organism responsible for the inflammation typical of acne.

─ **Pores**

The skin's opening is above the hair follicle.

─ **Pimple**

Another name for a papule.

— Pustule

Spherical, inflamed lesions that are typically filled with pus. They tend to progress and form more deep-penetrating nodules. Retinoid A chemical derived from vitamin A which is often used for treating moderate to severe acne.

— Scarring

A result of the body's natural healing process, scarring occurs when either too little tissue has been produced to reform the skin in a damaged area or too much collagen tissue is present as a result of over-assertive healing.

— Sebaceous Glands

The glands in the follicles which produce oils for lubricating the skin.

— Sebum

The oil produced by the sebaceous glands.

— Whitehead

A closed comedo, a non-inflammatory acne lesion.

— Zit

A slang word used for pimple.

How Acne Physically Develops

Acne usually first rears its ugly head during the teen years of a girl. The main reason for this is because of the onset of puberty and the hormones that are being released in the body at this time. **So, remember it is the hormones in the body that causes acne**, not the chocolate or greasy foods that they are eating. That is just a myth.

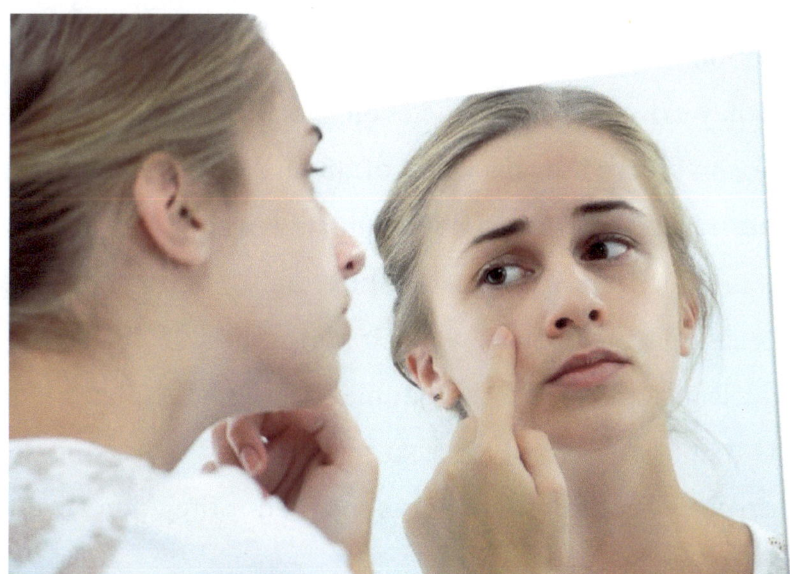

Once the body starts to produce hormones, it causes the oil glands in the skin to be overactive. This extra oil then will combine with the dead skin cells, and then the pores become clogged because of this. It is how the bacteria will get in and

get trapped and will then begin to irritate the skin and cause what we know as pimples, blackheads and whiteheads.

There are times when the pimples won't develop with a white head or blackhead and will swell and be a red and sometimes painful bump. Generally, though the blister will fill with pus and will be white-tipped, the common pimple that we all hate and dread.

The physical effects of acne manifest as red blotches and inflammations of the skin. The blemishes can sometimes get so bad that they can get infected and even, in the end, leave the skin of the person scarred for life. A lot of the unfortunate problems with acne, however, are from bad habits that a person has when it comes to their skincare. Some of those habits are when teens scrub their skin way too hard which irritates the skin even more, or they will pick at or pop the pimple. Using makeup and hair products that are oil-based are also a contributor to making the acne worse. These things should be avoided if they don't want the acne to spread.

Although most acne is not severe, some cases are and must be treated by a doctor. There is one type that generally is seen in males that are called acne fulminans.

It is rare and can even lead to fever and joints that ache. It can also cause weight to lose because the appetite is affected, and there is also high white blood count in the bloodstream. It can spread to the back and chest as well. This type of acne must always be treated by a doctor.

The psychological factors for a teen who has acne can be immense. Having a good social life for a teen is probably the essential thing in their lives, and nothing destroys that quicker than a super bad case of acne. The psychological effects of this can be devastating to some teens. They will begin to feel ugly or start thinking that other people believe that they are a dirty person. Acne adds more stress to a teens life, and this then can lead to even more acne breakouts.

Acne can be quite traumatic for a teen, especially if their parents don't seem to understand and are not sympathetic about this particular issue in their lives. It can lead to feelings of depression, as well as a sense of insecurity. A teen who has terrible acne can often not want to do anything socially and want to stay locked up at home.

Seeing how acne affects teenage girls the most according to studies, it can have a social impact on their lives. It is probably the most difficult to deal with at this age due to all the changes happening to your body, such as going through puberty. No matter how much pain and self-pity one feels, you have to remind yourself that acne is only temporary and can be dealt with.

Hyper Sensitivity towards Acne

Teenage girls tend to be much more sensitive to their appearance and the judgments of their peers. In adolescence, physical appearance conventionality tends to be highly valued, so those teenagers who suffer from acne may feel socially devalued and isolated from their peers. Even mild acne, research shows, can have an emotionally and psychologically devastating effect. Higher rates of anxiety, depression, and low self-esteem have all been linked with the presence of acne.

Because adolescence is a period of emotional sensitivity. Mild acne can cause significant emotional stress for a teenager. Most teenagers with acne tend to develop a negative self-image. It may lead to a withdrawal from friends and family.

Understanding the Cause of Acne

What are the causes of acne? Why are teen girls more susceptible to this condition?

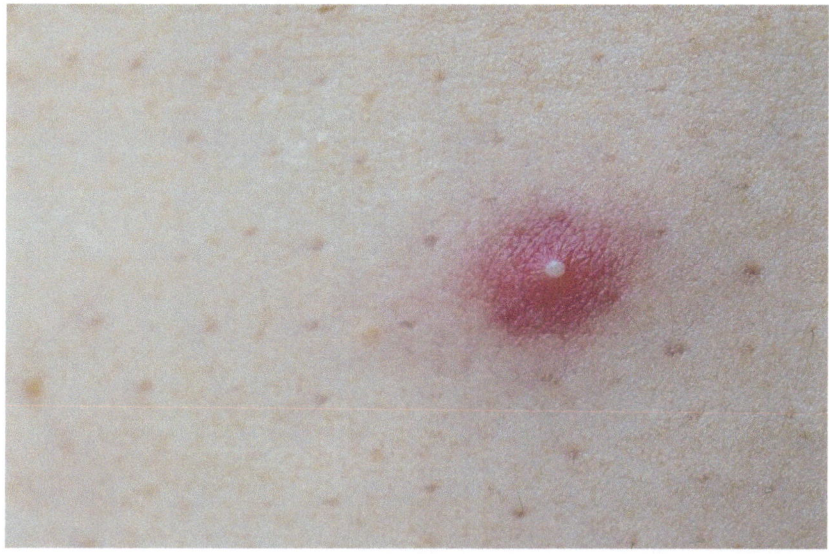

Acne is a prevalent dermatological condition which can be quite disfiguring and has longer-term effects. It tends to affect adolescent people but is by no means limited to them. What are the causes of acne? Find the answers in our report, learn about the underlying causes and read about some acne myths that we debunk, too.

A Dermatological Disaster

The basis for an acne outbreak lies in the blockage of hair follicles in the skin. The follicles and associated sebaceous glands usually produce a natural protein called keratin. They also shed dead skin cells from the follicle lining, and a natural oil called sebum. In acne, keratin and sebum are produced to excess. The follicles become blocked by keratin, sebum and dead skin cells. The blockages lead to the symptoms of acne.

Once the follicles (or pores) get blocked, a specific bacterium called Propionibacterium which is ordinarily harmless infects the blocked ducts. The result is inflammation and damage to the skin and underlying tissue. The bacterium (usually abbreviated to P. acnes) is anaerobic. It means that it does not use oxygen to survive. It does best in the absence of oxygen, so it's perfectly adapted to cause maximum trouble in blocked pores.

It's All In Your Hormones

Both genetic factors and the body's hormones are key issues when considering what the causes of acne are. The rate of keratin production is linked to genetic factors. This is why acne has a significant genetic dependency. In other words, it tends to run in families. Due to the presence of male hormones called androgens, the rate of sebum production increases in puberty.

The male sex hormones cause enlargement of the sebaceous glands and increase the speed of sebum production.

The effect on the skin's pores varies. They may be blocked, become enlarged and appear as blackheads, papules, pustules and so on. Some may become closed pockets of dead skin cells; these are a pervasive dermatological feature known as milia and are not limited to acne. In girls and women, hormonal changes linked to menstruation may also contribute to the likelihood of an acne outbreak.

Just for the record, the androgens that are associated with acne are testosterone, dihydrotestosterone (DHT) and dehydroepiandrosterone sulphate (DHEAS).

There's another similar cause which does not arise naturally - steroids. The use of anabolic steroids can lead to acne as they have a very same effect to naturally occurring androgens.

Although acne is frequently seen in adolescence and early adult life, it may break out later in life too. What are the causes of acne later on in life? Hormone activity naturally increases during pregnancy, and as a consequence, pregnant women are disposed to suffering acne outbreaks. During the menopause, there is a progressive reduction in the production of the female hormone estradiol, and acne is sometimes seen at this time as a result.

It is seen that many teen girls at school age suffer from acne due to family history, and they inherit this problem from their parents. Some of the other factors like bad eating habits, constipation and depression, can also cause acne. Certain medications like contraceptive pills and anti-psychotics also prove to aggravate the hormone changes causing acne breakouts in some people.

Other Causes Of Acne

There may be a relationship between stress and acne. Opinions do vary, but it is commonly proposed that an increase of pressure may provoke or worsen an acne outbreak. The causality is still disputed. Although there is a likely correlation between stress and acne, it is not clear if the fear results from the challenges of enduring acne, or the other way round.

What are the causes of acne that we might be able to deal with ourselves? Perhaps we could avoid acne by making changes to our diet. There is good evidence that a high GL diet tends to make acne worse. GL is glycemic load; it expresses how much carbohydrate is present in the food and its effect on the

levels of glucose in the blood. High GL food tends to cause towering peaks in blood glucose levels which may, in turn, worsen the severity of acne, amongst other undesirable effects.

And finally, the inflammation may spout into whiteheads, blackheads, pustules (commonly known as pimples or zits), or cysts. These factors are the answers to the question of what are the causes of acne.

The Factors That Increase Acne

Do you suffer from severe acne? Do you know the causes of your acne? Do you know how to cure them? Well, if you don't, then continue reading to learn more and have enough knowledge about the factors that increase acne

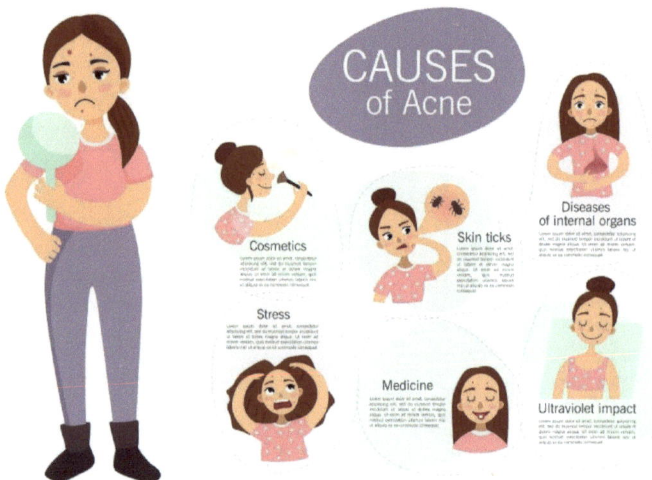

The real cause of acne is undetermined, but dermatologist believes that they result from numerous factors. Such factors include:

— Rising Of Hormone Levels

Growing in hormone level is one of the most critical factors. The androgen hormones, male sex hormones, increase in girls during their teenage years.

During these years, the sebaceous gland enlarges and produces more sebum. Once more sebum is created; the pores get clogged with oil, and then acne starts to occur.

— Changing Of Hormone Levels

Women and younger girls (particularly adolescents) can cause a flare-up in their pimples or acne two to seven days before the start of their menstrual period.

Moreover, the hormones of women change during pregnancy, and when they stop using birth control pills, this can be another cause of acne.

— Picking and Squeezing

It is common to see that acne sufferers pick at the acne lesions and squeeze out the retained sebaceous deposits. And it is a commonly mistaken impression that this will unblock the pore and speed up healing.

The squeezing cause unnecessary damage to the skin; bacteria are introduced to the wound and causes inflammation. The result is often darker, deeper and more permanent scars.

− Stress

Acne gets worse when the person suffers from fear, worry, tension and anxiety. For example, it has been observed that during the examination period, the acne condition get worse for student suffers. It is likely to cause by hormones and neuroactive substances produced during stress and significantly influence on acne formation.

− Premenstrual Flares

Some girls complain of acne flares just before their menses. And these premenstrual flares affect up to 40% of girls with acne.

It is likely due to the hormone fluctuation over the menstrual cycle. The flares often resolve quickly after the end of the menses.

− Creams and Medication

Certains cosmetics and medication may make acne worse. Topical steroids which are often prescribed for treating eczema may result in an outbreak of acne is they are used excessively and inappropriately.

You can identify this type of acne by its look - multiple red, inflamed monomorphic papules and pustules.

─ Drugs

Some drugs aggravate or even cause acne. These include:

- Corticosteroids which are taken orally or by injections
- Lithium for treating manic depressive illness
- Testosterone pills and injection which are used by professional athletes and bodybuilders to increase muscle mass
- Danazol which is given to women for endometriosis which is the growth of tissue from the uterus in parts of the body other than the uterus

─ Cosmetics

For a small group of cosmetics users, they can develop cosmetic acne in the form of side effect.

Cosmetic acne is usually present as small, raised whiteheads or small inflamed papules and pustules over the face the cosmetics are applied.

Often, women with superficial acne are caught in a vicious cycle - the more acne outbreak they have, the more cosmetics up they use to cover it up, which only leads to worsening of the condition.

— Climate

Acne tends to get worse in hot, humid climates and work environment, e.g. steam rooms and kitchen. We do not know why heat and humidity have such an aggravating effect, but we know is that the outer layer of skin swells tremendously under humid conditions. The pressure from the swelling could block the opening of the pilosebaceous unit and cause acne to develop.

— Friction

The friction caused by rubbing, leaning on and the pressure from your tight collars, backpacks, and bike helmets do contribute in the worsening of your acne.

So, these are the factors that increases acne to re-occur in teen girls.

Conventional Treatment with Their Side Effects

When you want to find out what is the best acne treatment, you should first look at the track record of the conventional acne treatments prescribed by dermatologists. These are antibiotics and Accutane, both of which are proven to clear up acne to some degree, although they are very limited in the results they get.

The first problem with both antibiotics and Accutane is that if they work, they only work for a short period, usually just weeks or months. Once they stop working, they become useless in treating acne. The second problem is that they have adverse side effects.

It is the most potent and effective acne medication in the whole world. It's beneficial because it reduces the production of sebum or facial oil. Without much facial fat, the pores on your skin will not get clogged, and as a result, acne cannot form. While this is an effective zit zapper, but Accutane does cause many severe side effects.

Some of these side effects include:

- Your lips get dried as soon as you take the pill.

- Your kidney and liver have to work at

Antibiotics are shown to cause candida, which is an infestation of harmful bacteria which causes many health problems such as fatigue. While Accutane's most common side effect is depression, a mental condition that makes one feel emotionally sad most of the time. When deciding what the best acne treatment is, you should weigh up the positive (clear skin for a limited time) with the negative (unwanted side effects.)

The conventional acne treatments described above are generally considered to be the weakest if somewhat more predictable acne treatments around. But when asking what the best acne treatment is, you need to be aware of more natural acne treatments available that don't have side effects.

These come in two general types; acne cleansers and pills explicitly made to treat acne (examples include proactive, Murad and Zen med), and natural acne treatment programs designed specifically for clearing acne (cases include Acne Free in 3 Days, Acne No More and Mr. X Acne Says.) The benefits of using cleansers and pills made for treating acne is that they are usually straightforward to use every day, require a simple action of cleansing with a particular product once or twice a day, or popping a few pills.

The drawback of these acne cleansers and pills is that they are expensive and require repeated purchases every month or two, and have a poor track record of working effectively. The benefits of using an acne cure program are that they work on treating acne holistically, which not only improves acne but general health as well. The drawback is that they require more effort than simply popping a few pills, and need a certain amount of commitment to get acne-clearing results.

So, what are the most common treatments for acne? To list just a few, they are:

- Benzoyl Peroxide
- Accutane
- Topical antibiotics
- Oral antibiotics

The Ugly Truth About Benzoyl Peroxide

Most pimple products on sale in the market today are benzoyl peroxide-based. Benzoyl peroxide can kill the acne-causing bacteria and dry up your skin to "speed up the healing of the zits." It is decently effective for light acne, but not so when it comes to more severe types of acne. So, should you use benzoyl peroxide-based creams or lotions? I don't think so.

The worse thing about benzoyl peroxide is that it causes excessive irritation and dryness. If any of these happens, your skin will painfully hurt. These side effects occur more common than you might think.

For the first few weeks or months of using benzoyl peroxide, you will probably not feel any of these adverse side effects. But BP products need to be used

continually to be effective. As you continue the treatment, your skin will become thinner and thinner and more susceptible to UV rays and irritations.

The Acne & Blood Sugar

Acne is caused by an increase in skin cell turnover and excess sebum blocking the pores of the skin. This then leads to bacteria flourishing at the site of the blocked pore and creating inflammation. The causes of this are somewhat complicated; however, here, we will be discussing how high levels of blood sugar contribute to the problem in teen girls.

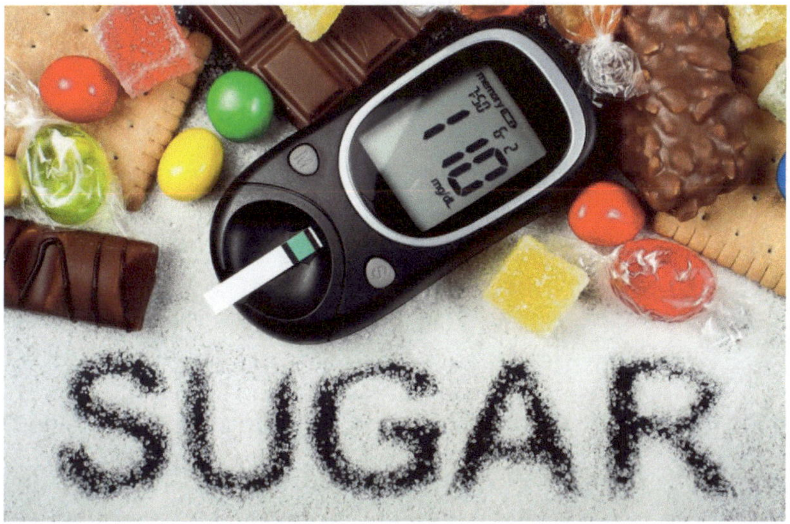

Several scientific studies have shown that people with acne do not process sugar properly. It is this connection between high blood sugar and acne that led two scientists to call acne "skin diabetes."

When we eat carbohydrates, they are digested into individual glucose molecules. These are then absorbed from the gut into the bloodstream where they can enter our cells and be burned for energy. When sugar is released into the bloodstream, the pancreas is triggered to release the hormone insulin, which transports the sugar into our cells. People with acne have been shown to do this ineffectively.

The level of sugar that is in the bloodstream at any one time can be affected by the types of carbohydrates we eat. Some carbohydrates are broken down into glucose molecules quicker than others. The rate at which a carb does this can be measured by what's called its Glycaemic Load (GL). A food with a high GL, such as 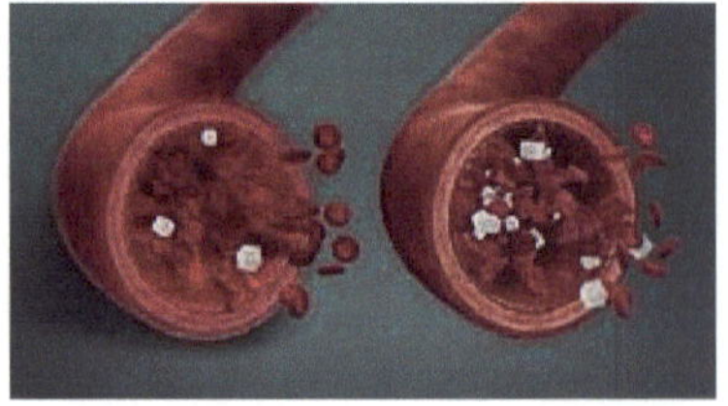 sugar or refined carbohydrates, releases its sugar quickly, whereas one with a low GL has a slower release.

When we overeat of food with a high GL, this causes a large amount of sugar to be dumped into the bloodstream, which then triggers a large amount of insulin to remove it. Eating in this way, as well as consuming stimulants such as coffee, tea and alcohol, which also raise the blood sugar, can lead to the cells becoming resistant to insulin. When this happens, insulin is unable to do its job of transporting sugar into the cells effectively. In response to this, the body then produces even more insulin to try to lower the blood sugar.

The problem with high insulin for acne sufferers is that insulin does more than merely lower blood sugar. When in high amounts, it can trigger sebum and skin cell production as well as leading to hormone imbalances which are also found in acne sufferers.

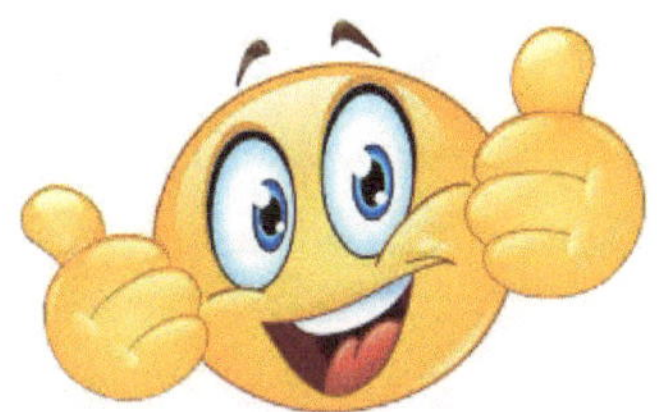 It, therefore, makes sense, in trying to get rid of acne, to follow a low GL diet to reduce insulin output. However, there are several other factors which control insulin levels different than your Glycaemic load. There are also other causes of acne other than your blood sugar. The good news is that all of these can be taken care of with natural methods. The first step, however, would be to manage your blood sugar with a low GL diet.

How Does Your Diet And Your Blood Type Affect Your Health?

Now imagine that a Type "O." You belong to the high-protein meat-eaters diet profile. Your body will only tolerate legumes, grains and beans in lesser quantities. So, if you find yourself on a vegetarian diet, your body is going to react negatively. Some proteins found in your food causes this reaction.

These proteins are called lectins. Your genetic makeup as an O blood type means that these lectins are going to keep you healthy only if you eat lots of meat. The moment you start eating a vegetarian diet and cut down on the meat, the lectins are going to harm your blood, on a particular organ in your body or on your general system. However, you do not have to worry about these lectins being very dangerous; the body's natural immunity system is capable of protecting your body against their potentially harmful agglutinating effect on your blood cells.

98% of these lectins are removed from your body during its natural elimination processes.

Nevertheless, your diet is going to affect your health. That, in turn, is going to hurt your skin. That is why you might see your skin breaking out in acne.

How does Your Blood Type Affect An Acne Outbreak?

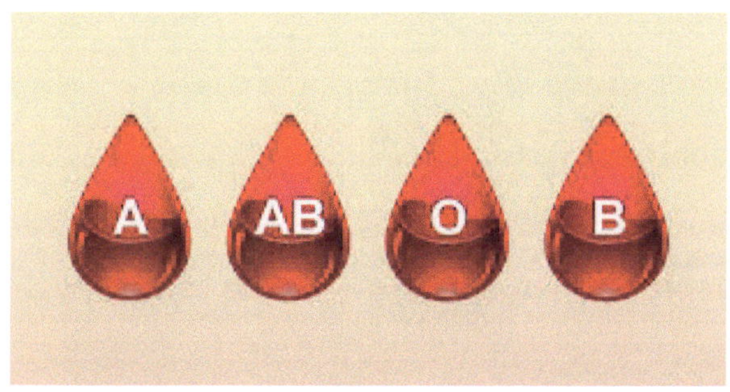

Each blood type has several foods which are helpful, beneficial and medicinal for it. These are the foods which are best suited to a person's genetic inheritance and which are best tolerated by her body. On the other hand, there are several foods which are going to harm one's body, depending on her blood type.

Also, each blood type has a tolerance level for many foods which have a neutral effect on the blood type.

Now imagine that you are a type A which has a vegetarian and seafood genetic inheritance. You thrive on grains, legumes, seafood, vegetables and fruit. Meat, wheat and dairy products are not beneficial for you. Now, suppose you find yourself eating a diet with plenty of meat in it.

It is going to hurt your body's bio-physiological processes. You may find yourself suffering a lot from acne. So, you need to clear your system by switching to a fruit and vegetable diet as well as increase the number of grains and legumes in your daily meals.

A type B is omnivorous and can eat meat without any chicken, beans, cereals, fruit and vegetables, which are healing and beneficial foods. However, if they begin to eat a diet rich in seeds, chicken, tomatoes, and shellfish, they are going to find themselves suffering from ill-health. They are also going to find themselves suffering from potential acne outbreaks.

So, if you are suffering from acne, it is a good idea to find out your blood type. After that, start eating the foods which are best suited to your genetic makeup and inheritance. It is going to keep you healthy. It is also going to give you a glowing skin free of acne, blackheads, whiteheads and pimples.

Acne & Fatty Foods

Acne, the word itself is enough to give nightmares to any person, especially the teenage girls. What if we tell you that the food you consume is also responsible for your problem to a certain extent? Some food items when eaten can cause and even aggravate this problem, and if you try to avoid these foods, you can reduce acne and also get rid of them.

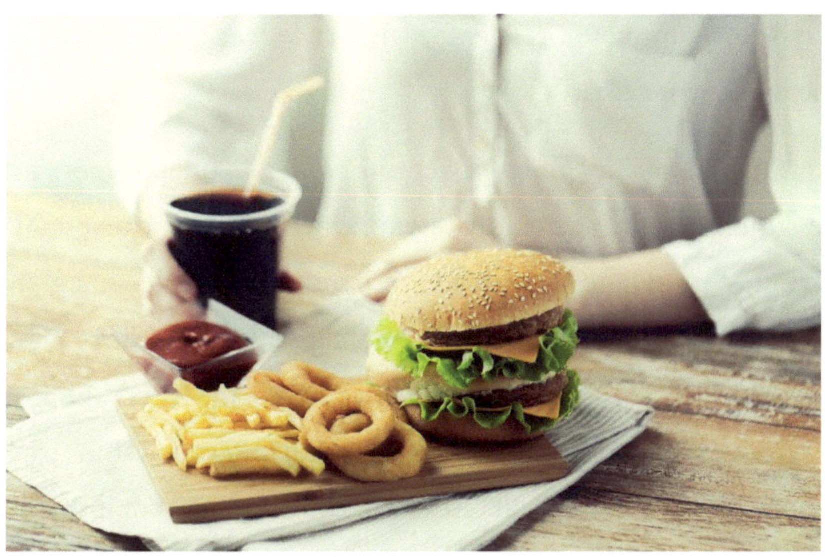

Do Fatty Foods Cause Acne?

It is a question that many people have been pondering over for years. Some people assume that it does, while a few others consider it as a myth. For some, it is a doubt that lingers around. Perhaps, you too have come across various rumours about fat and acne.

But, can you imagine cutting out pizza, ice-creams, French fries and chocolates from your diet? That is if they are your favourite snacks! Let's go on to discuss this matter in detail.

Imagine a teenage girl gulping down several servings of fried chicken and waking up the next day with red bulges over his skin. Are the zits related to fatty food? Until recently, the answer would have been a 'no,' but today, studies suggest that there 'maybe' a connection. The fat you eat does not directly re-emerge on your skin.

But it stimulates hormonal reactions, which in turn triggers acne breakouts. You're probably aware that acne is caused by a hormonal imbalance that leads to overactive sebaceous glands in your skin. The excess oil or sebum secreted by these glands clogs the skin pores, allowing bacterial growth. The response of your immune system inflames the portion and causes bumps. So, what you eat matters. And fatty foods affect your skin indirectly.

Being the largest organ of your body, your skin is prone to some sort of influence by the foods you consume. What exactly happens when too much fat is ingested? When you consume fatty and oily foods or sugary foods, the pancreas produces more insulin. This, in turn, leads to increased secretion of androgen, a male hormone that is responsible for hyperactivity of the sebaceous glands. It results in excessive sebum production, and so on. We just discussed it in the previous paragraph.

What kind of fats should you avoid? Fat is a nutrient required by your body, and hence, you cannot deprive your body of an essential nutrient. It is only when you consume too much of it that you face a problem. Saturated fats are considered as unhealthy fats, as they distress your immune system, increase inflammation and trigger the oil glands. They are linked to other health disorders, including heart problems. On the other hand, healthy fats contained in fish oil, flax oil and olive oil have anti-inflammatory properties that are good for your body.

Pay attention to your diet as a whole and avoid overly spicy, greasy, fatty and processed foods, which increase your hormone production and trigger the oil glands. During your teens, your body is already under the influence of hormonal changes, so you must make up your mind to adopt a balanced diet and a healthy lifestyle. Your genetics and skin type are indeed essential factors that decide the intensity of your acne.

But you can have control provided you are ready to learn certain healthy habits. There are acne vitamins and natural remedies that are known to give positive results.

It just takes a little effort on your part to examine the kinds of food you consume and the type of lifestyle you pursue. **Ultimately, a balanced diet, a good exercise regime, sufficient sleep and other healthy habits will boost your overall health and also keep you acne-free.**

Stay Away From These Foods

Start with controlling your intake of foods rich in oil and fats like mayonnaise, butter and some salad dressings. They are very pleasing both to our taste buds and to our eyes but are very bad for health and increase acne. To get rid of acne, you have to stay away from oily, greasy and fatty foods.

Sugar, baked goods, processed flour, sweets and hydrogenated or trans fats are the food items that again play a significant role in increasing acne. These are available in foods like donuts, cookies, pastry, pies, etc. You must try not to eat cakes, loaves of bread, and chips regularly as they promote acne. Avoid the use of any sodas. They are unhealthy and increase acne. Foods rich in carbohydrates are known to produce a high glycemic load, which causes a rise in blood sugar or the insulin levels in the blood. Excess oil builds up under the skin and pore blockages can occur due to higher levels of insulin. So, avoid sugared drinks, white bread and white potatoes etc. that are a rich source of carbohydrates.

Limit the intake of milk products like ice cream, cheese etc. These products, especially the ones made from cow's milk, are rich in hormones. If the liquid is from a pregnant cow, then the hormone level will be even higher. These products, when consumed, get broken down into dihydrotestosterone (DHT), which again turns into the oil making cells. Elimination of milk and milk products will undoubtedly improve the acne problem.

Limit the intake of nuts like pistachio, walnuts, and hazelnuts etc. These kinds of nuts and even peanuts and peanut butter also provoke acne. The best way to deal with acne is an acne prevention diet. Though trying to control acne is very difficult, but a little diet control and diet planning can help a lot. Here are a few easy tips for you:

- The easiest and most effective way to cleanse your body is by drinking lots of water. Consume lots of water instead of sodas and try herbal teas and vegetable juices.

- Instead of sugar, you can take no-calorie sweeteners.

- Avoid all types of fatty foods.

- Switch to more complex carbohydrates with fibre, for example, unrefined beans or cereals. These foods have a low glycemic index, and so they help in reducing acne.

- Reduce the intake of milk and milk products.

This kind of diet may not be able to cure your acne problem entirely, but it will reduce or limit the number of foods that can aggravate your case of acne. It will make your skin healthier and will reduce the amount of acne that appears on your surface.

Natural Treatment for Acne

The best natural treatment for acne problem is choosing the type of food you take. A correctly formulated diet can help your body to eliminate toxins and waste effectively, so it does not have the chance to remain in your body and cause acne. **To cure acne problems, it has to start from the inside out. That means it has to start from within your organization.**

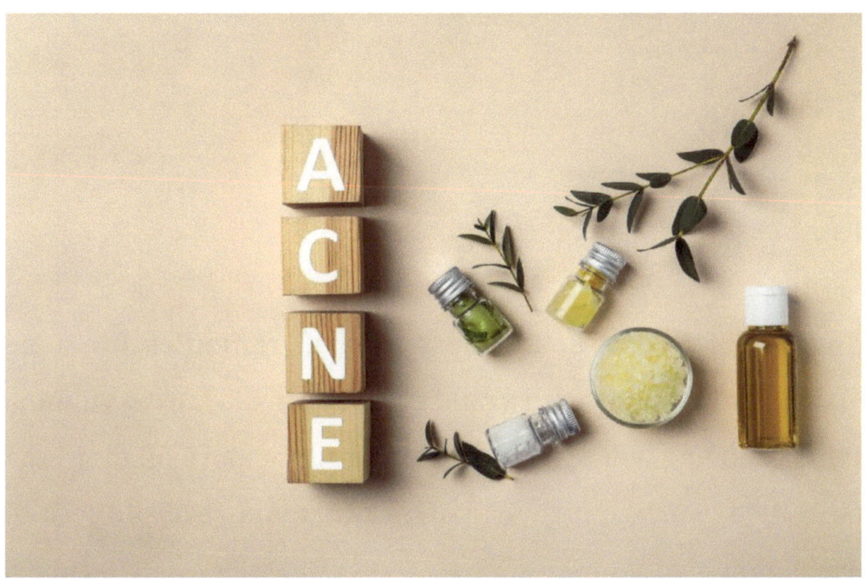

You've tried scrubbing it, covering it up, and applying expensive goo by the jarful. Now you're ready to go in a different direction to get rid of that acne. There are natural remedies for acne that work, and that may also improve your overall health.

The excess production of natural oils causes acne. So, you want to take steps to dry the oil, but you don't want to dry it too much. It will create a rebound effect, and your skin will produce more oil in response. Here are some products you can apply to your skin that will provide natural remedies for acne without drying it too much:

- Witch hazel
- Tree oil
- Aloe Vera
- Honey
- Oatmeal
- Avocado (mixed with water)

Cleanliness is one of the best natural remedies for acne. Wash your face daily with a mild soap, and avoid hard scrubbing. Hard scrubbing will make your skin produce more oil to protect itself. Also, wash your hair daily, as this will result in less oil production near your face.

Make sure that everything that comes near your face is clean all the time. Keep your hats, coats, scarves, shirts, ties, hair bands, glasses, and so forth clean. Make sure your bedding, such as your blanket and pillowcase, is clean. Also, avoid touching your face.

A healthy lifestyle is an excellent natural remedy for acne. Watch what you eat. The old wives' tale is accurate; oily and sugary foods will contribute to acne. _Eat plenty of fruits and vegetables and drink green tea. Fruits, vegetables, and green tea contain antioxidants that are powerful against acne. Get plenty of exercises. The improved circulation you get from use is perfect for your skin._

Try to exercise outdoors, since sunlight is an excellent natural astringent (be careful to avoid sunburn, though).

Get plenty of sleep and drink a lot of water, as these will give you energy and help you get through your day with less stress. Stress is a great contributor to acne.

Find some quiet time for yourself each day to help reduce stress.

─ Carrots

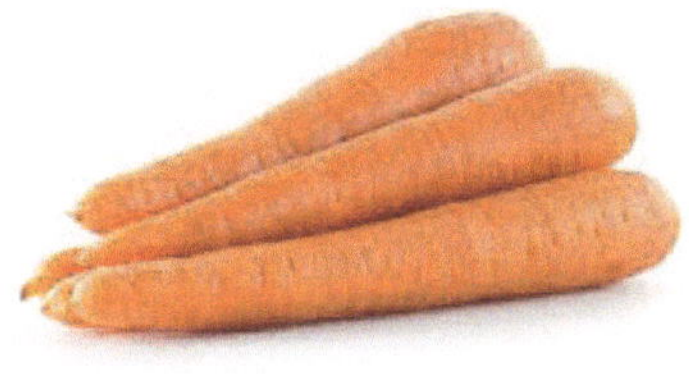

You might wonder why carrots can help you in fighting acne. Well, carrots are full of vitamin-A, and vitamin-A are useful for reducing the production of your sebum or natural body oil. As you might know, one factor that causes the development of acne is because of excessive production of body oil. So, by consuming vitamin- A and your sebum production reduced, you can avoid worsening your condition.

─ Natural yogurt

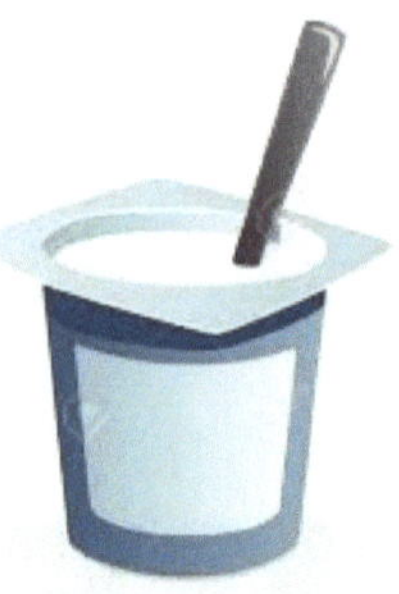

It is also useful as natural treatments for acne because yogurt can be used to clear your pores that have become blocked by dead skin cells. One reason why you have acne is that your pores are clogged and this prevents your sebum from escaping freely, so keep your pores clean are a good idea.

Before spending a lot of time and money on acne treatments, try these natural remedies for acne. You may find that not only has your acne improved, you feel better as well.

Essential Oils for Acne

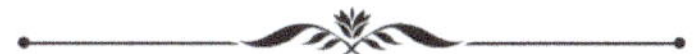

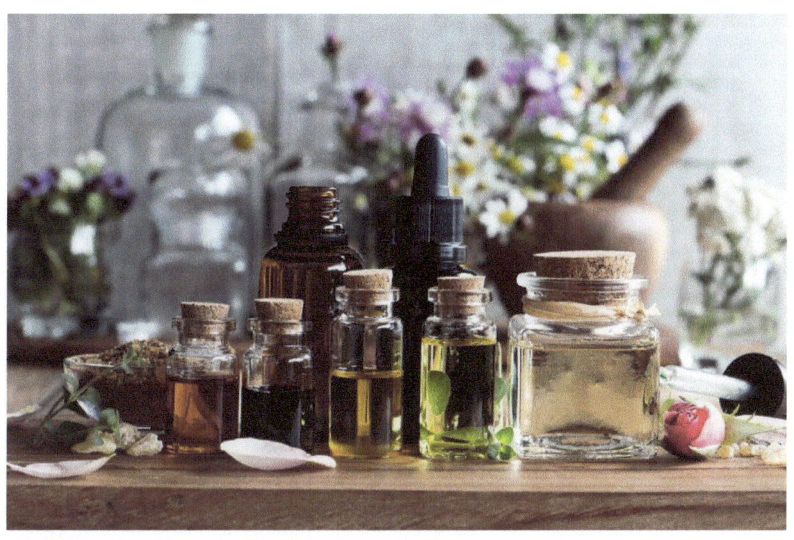

Can essential oils be an effective acne treatment? The answer is Yes, but you will need a little patience with it.

Essential oils are concentrated distillations of various plants (including the flower, stalks, leaves and roots) and many have anti-fungal, anti-bacterial and anti- inflammatory properties. For those who want a more holistic and natural approach to acne and acne scar treatment, this may be the answer or part of a solution to your problems. First of all, you will need to find out which plant or flower oils are best for you. Even with specific essential oils for acne and acne scars, everyone will react differently, so it is best to spend some time to find the best one for you. Essential oils for acne is, therefore, a very personal experience.

A few safety notes:

- If you are ill, check with your doctor first as some essential oils can be dangerous for specific conditions.

- Essential oils (except for lavender and rose oil) needs to be applied to a base or carrier oil before application. The recommended dosage is 12-15 drops of essential oil to one ounce of carrier oil.

- Do not rub the oils into your eyes or ingest them internally.

The best essential oils for skincare can be used for many different applications, including:

- As an acne fighter

- As an astringent for clearing away dead skin

- To soothe and help heal chapped or cracked skin

- For mild cleansing

- To revitalize you, by adding certain minerals or vitamins found in the oils

- To moisturize dry skin

- To moisturize eczema and help soothe it

- To help alleviate itching, inflammation, and possible infections

- To help smooth out wrinkles and make you look younger

So, with that out of the way, let us look at some of these high natural oils:

─ **Lavender**

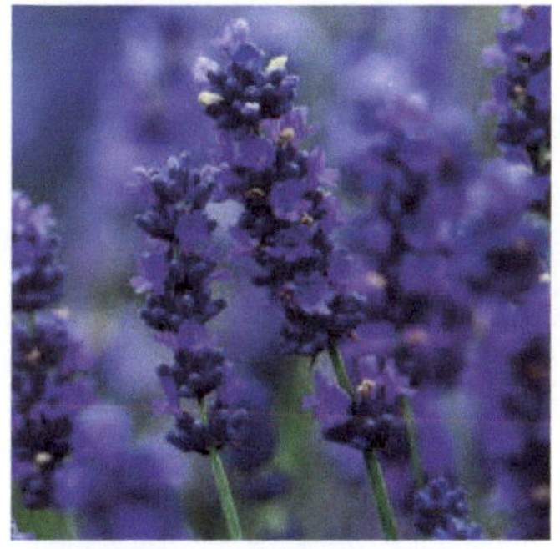

Lavender is probably the most used and most versatile essential oil. It is also one of the only oils you can apply directly onto your skin without a carrier oil. It has all the anti-bacterial properties to combat infections and has been used for centuries as an antiseptic.

Applied directly onto spots, it will reduce inflammation and kill off bacteria. A lavender water spray is also an excellent way to refresh your face.

For sufferers of body acne, a few drops in a bath will help reduce outbreaks.

─ Geranium

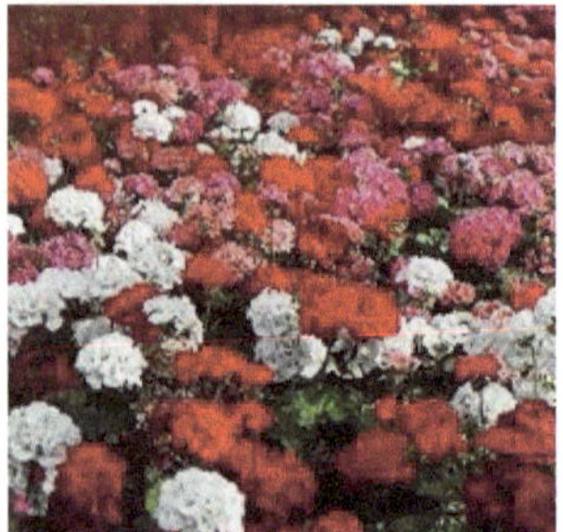

Geranium has excellent balancing properties and is the right choice to restore your skin to its natural state, whether it is too dry or too oily.

It has a delightful aroma and mixes well with most other oils such as rose and jasmine.

─ Bergamot

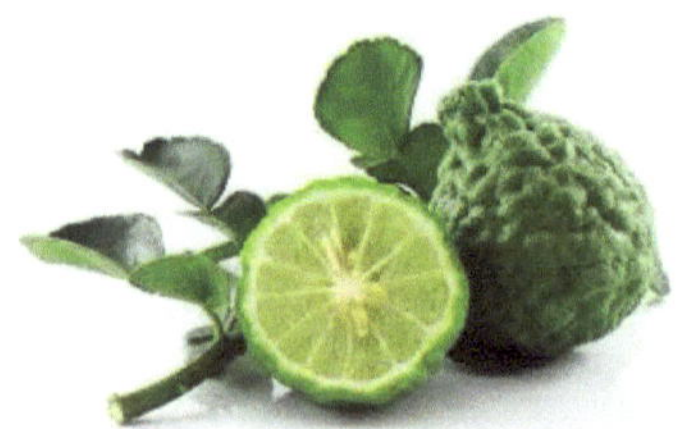

Bergamot has a citrus fragrance found in Earl Grey tea. Light and fresh, bergamot has drying and anti-bacterial properties that are effective in combating skin breakouts.

Be careful, though when using bergamot as it makes the skin more sensitive to the sun's rays.

─ Clove

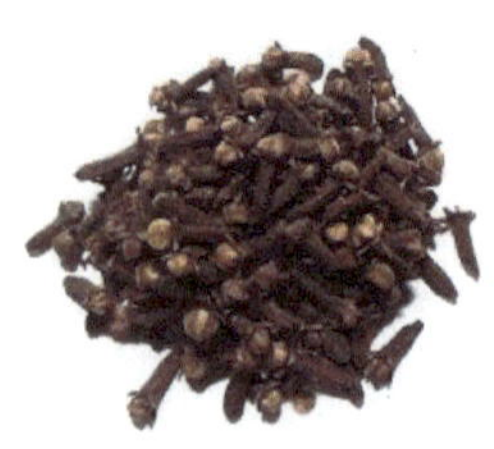

Clove, on the other hand, is quite active in both aromas and its healing properties.

Even though it has strong anti-fungal and anti-inflammatory properties, it is not advisable to apply it directly onto the skin also though it has been used to treat more stubborn acne. If you are not sure about Clove, try a small amount first.

⎯ Tea Tree

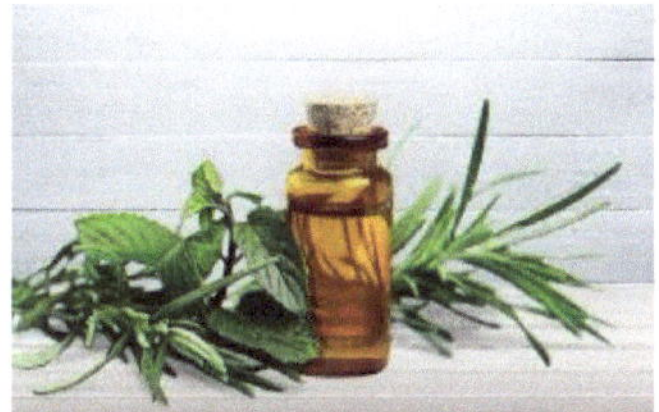

Tea tree oil is well known for its healing and anti-bacterial properties. It heals wounds, soothes rashes, gets rid of dandruff, soothes burns and stops infections. As an essential oil to combat acne, tea tree's anti-bacterial and other properties are very useful. It will also prevent irritation and calm inflammations.

⎯ Rosewood

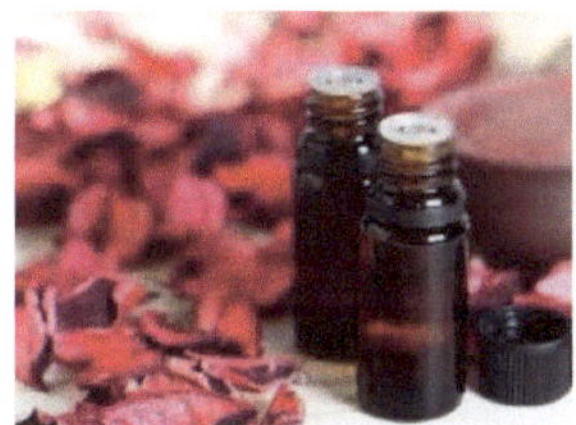

Rosewood oil has strong drying abilities and is best used for oily skin. It can dry out individual spots and breakouts, but if you have healthy or dry skin, you should avoid using it in other areas.

⎯ Carrier Oils

The best type of carrier or base oil is those using the "cold press" method. The oils are extracted naturally without using any healing process, which means the natural properties of the oils are not distorted.

— Rosemary Oil

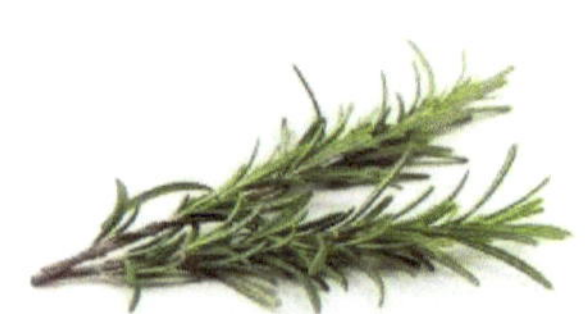

Rosemary oil is an often-overlooked herb that also does wonders for revitalizing skin, besides adding flavour in the kitchen! It's well known for its abilities to reduce excess oil on the surface. Besides, it also contains anti-inflammatory properties known to ease redness and puffiness, which is perfect for treating breakouts. Besides helping to clear skin, rosemary also improves circulation, which can help firm and tone. It's a versatile oil that makes a great addition to your beauty routine.

— Frankincense Oil

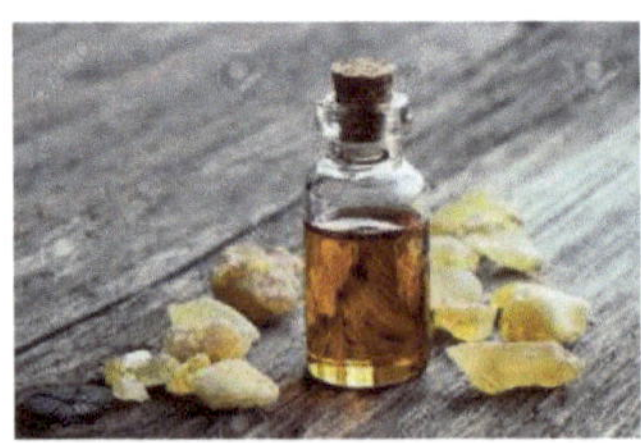

Frankincense oil is another oil great for acne-prone skin. This oil acts in an anti-bacterial and anti-inflammatory way. It is known as a healing and therapeutic oil, in addition to battling pimples effectively. It also acts as a natural toner and tightens the skin, reducing wrinkles and scars, so it may be able to do double-duty as an acne fighter and anti-ager!

— Oregano Oil

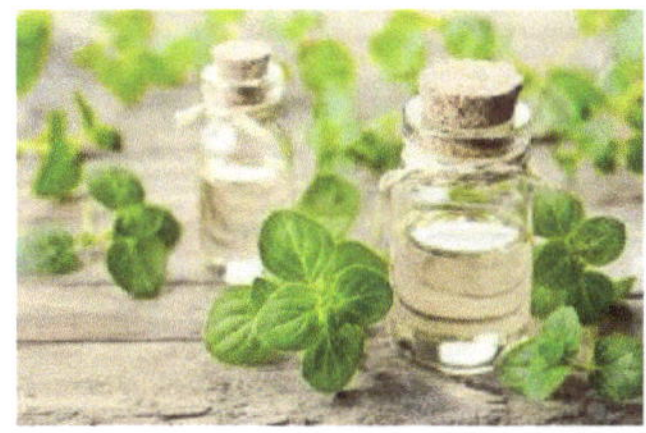 Not just amazing in the kitchen, oregano in its essential oil form is also fantastic for getting rid of pimples. The natural antiseptic and antibacterial properties of oregano oil make it handy for spot treating zits. As with the other oils, oil of oregano has amazing anti-bacterial properties. It also has many different uses, notably being used to prevent colds.

— Ylang Ylang Oil

The ylang-ylang essential oil comes from the flowers of a tropical tree (Cananga odorata) native to South-East Asia. Ylang ylang is also very popular for its a lovely floral scent but is also used in a variety of applications, particularly aromatherapy and perfumery.

In traditional herbal medicine, ylang-ylang oil was used extensively in topical treatments for skin and hair problems. The oil was also to have calming and anti- pyretic (anti-fever) properties. Ylang-ylang oil also has a positive effect on skin tone and can improve oily skin.

There are many carrier oils, but for acne treatment, it all depends on your skin type.

- Greasy Oily Skin: Grape Seed, Almond and Apricot oils

- Healthy Skin: Jojoba, Calendula and Sesame

- Dry Skin: Wheat germ, Olive and Avocado

— Blending

Use a dark glass bottle (not plastic), and you could blend some of the essential's oils yourself with your favourite carrier oil. Combinations such as lavender with geranium, geranium with bergamot, all go quite well together.

Essential Oils for Acne Treatment

— Spot Treatment

Best used with: Tea Tree oil or Oregano Oil

How to do it:

Tea Tree Oil: You can place your tea tree oil on acne undiluted (once again, it is always recommended you do a skin test first) or mix a few drops of tea tree oil with Aloe Vera gel.

Apply to the affected area 1-2 times per day. If your skin tends to be dry, you should dilute the oil as tea tree oil can dry out your skin quickly.

Oregano Oil: It's best to dilute oregano oil before putting it on your face. Mix equal parts oregano oil and a carrier oil, like jojoba, olive or coconut oil. Then, dab the diluted mixture onto the trouble spot regularly until your skin clears up.

─ Create Your Own Facial Oil (Moisturizing!)

Best used with: Any of the above oils.

How to do it:

Pick out your favourite carrier oil (this could be coconut oil, jojoba oil, argan oil or even olive oil - though I'd recommend coconut!). Then choose your preferred essential oil and add around 4-7 drops. Do this slowly, mixing or shaking the container your oil is in. The scent should be detectable, but not overpowering.

Then, you're done!

The more you use essential oils for acne or any other areas of your life, the more ideas you will get for its uses. Before you know it, essential oils will become an integral part of your daily life.

Mistakes That Most Girls Make When Trying To Cure Acne Naturally

If you want to know what mistakes that usually girls make when they want to lose acne naturally then you have to read this chapter because you will discover those mistakes that prevent them from naturally cure their acne. From this, you should know what mistakes girls made, and you know what you should avoid or do for you to be able to cure acne naturally.

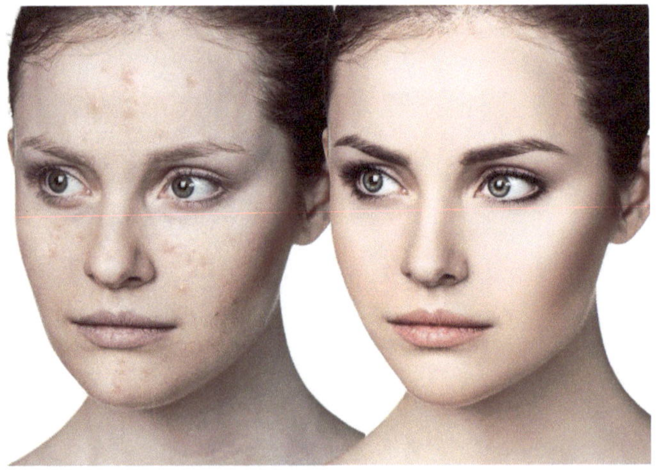

— They do not do a healthy diet

One of the natural remedies for acne is by doing a balanced diet, which means you change your habit from eating oily food to healthier food such as vegetables and fruits. Failed to do this and not only your body will be less healthy, but your body abilities on fighting bacteria that caused acne from inside can also be diminished. And this will make your effort on fighting acne will be much harder.

─ They do not take vitamins or take too many vitamins

Vitamin can also help your body fighting acne from inside. A specific dose of vitamins can help your body to fight acne. For example, by taking a small dose of vitamin-A, you can lower your body oil production if your body oil production reduced your face will not get dirty quickly.

What most girls do wrong is they take too many vitamins, this is not good for your body; you have to take vitamins sufficiently and do not go overboard it won't help you a bit.

─ They do not drink a lot of water

This one is another common mistake; they do not realize how important water is. Our body is 60% water, and knowing this, you should recognize the importance of water for our body. So, you might ask: "why water can help cure acne naturally?"

Water is a critical component in natural remedy for acne, water can help your body to flush out toxin that trigger acne from inside your body and also water is needed by your body in order for it to work correctly so if you give a lot of water to your body, you will make your body system function properly and fight acne from inside in the same time.

— They do not follow the right guide

One of the biggest mistakes that girls made is the failure to find a manual that can help them to cure acne naturally.

Final Remarks

As teen girls hit puberty and become a teenager, facial skincare becomes a critical factor for them, and it can affect their self-esteem.

Teenage girls are more concerned about their acne problems since it affects how they look. They always try to adopt new acne methods which would help them in reducing their acne problems. It also would sometimes lead them to have a worse skin condition.

As a result, they would have a loss of self-esteem and confidence. For them to have attractive skin, they need to adopt specific acne blemish control methods mentioned in this book and control the problem of deterioration of the surface.

Just like any other problem within the body, acne can only really be cured by removing the cause.

The successful curing of acne does not take place overnight, and for a teenage girl who wants miracle cures, this is not acceptable. So, parents should guide the teenager in this regard.

In conclusion, part of growing up means going through puberty. Puberty means acne, and that means having to deal with what we all deal with. Acne is something no one wants, but most of us get, especially teenage girls. Thankfully, acne in adolescent girls can be dealt with by eliminating fast and junk food from the diet. It is possible to have little or no acne as a teenager, but it means being proactive and not allowing yourself to eat bad foods. Also getting sunshine can help as well to stimulate the skin and help remove bacteria.

To your health,

Jerome Ohana.

NATURO-THERAPIST

About The Author

As a teenager, wanting to help others, he decided to take first aid training in case of emergency

This experience awakened in him to go further on the problems of health and their solutions: the conventional medicine approach (eliminated the disease) in comparison with alternative medicine (regenerated organism).

- Realized with time that nature had its own tradition of healing but yet unknown to the public due to the pharmacology system that surrounds us since our childhood.

He decided to take a courses in alternative medicine. chinese medicine health advisor health educator health practitioner (Naturo-therapist)

Today,

-Certified in Naturo-therapist by the "College Des Médecines Douce du Quebec"

-Certified in first aid responder by Hatzoloh Montreal organisation

He is waiting for one thing, to do his best to improve and generate people's health.